Expect
a Miracle

You Won't
Be Disappointed!

A Workbook for Your
Healing Journey
Using Appreciative Dialogue

TEL FRANKLIN, M.D.

Expect a Miracle . . . You Won't Be Disappointed!
A Workbook for Your Healing Journey
Using Appreciative Dialogue
by Tel Franklin

ISBN 0-9701165-0-0

Printed in the United States of America
Editor: Ann West
Jacket: Ben Cziller
Design: Kedron Bryson

PUBLISHED BY
CENTER FOR APPRECIATIVE DIALOGUE
335 El Dorado Street, Suite 6 • Monterey, California 93940
www.AppreciativeDialogue.org

My parents taught me that with discipline,
dedication and desire all dreams are
possibilities yet to be realized . . .
and most of all, that unconditional love
brings inner peace, which transforms all life.

To the memory of my brother Roger ~
lost in a second,
but who will be missed forever.

A Note to the Reader

Expect a Miracle . . . You Won't Be Disappointed! is not intended as medical advice. Its intent is solely informational and educational. Please consult a health care professional for specific treatments.

Appreciative Dialogue is an interactive workbook designed for individuals and health care practitioners. It acts as an adjunct to—not a substitute for—conventional allopathic medicine. When acute or chronic complaints (such as chest pain, headache, or back pain) are present, an appropriate diagnostic medical plan should be explored before seeking complementary modalities.

Be aware that any symptom may be an important sign of a potentially life-threatening situation, and all solutions (including natural remedies, manual therapy, and conventional medicine) should be postponed until after a thorough medical evaluation. Further, all treatment plans need to be individualized and closely monitored. Specific modalities—whether conventional or alternative—do not affect everyone in the same way. Some may not work for you, so please use caution. Partner with a physician who is knowledgeable and trustworthy, and critically scrutinize all suggested protocols.

Names of patients used in this work are fictitious; details of patients' histories are a synthesis of representative histories, and any resemblance to actual persons is entirely coincidental.

CONTENTS

Preface

This book comes from a spirit that has unleashed a passion at the core of my being. I feel driven to share a new path for viewing and accessing health care. Yet, this is not solely my book. It is a gift from all the experiences and teachers who have touched my life, especially my patients and the many pioneers in the field of complementary medicine.

Despite all the advances of medicine, modern allopathic care remains very limited; moreover, few practitioners initiate options. Instead, this book is about choices, a truly alternative approach to the healing arts. I invite you to use its dynamic process as a living resource to fulfill your goals and aspirations. From your inner self, it will reflect the life you deserve—and will make possible the highest quality of human health.

Appreciative Dialogue enables physicians to look at the world through the eyes of their patients. To that end, physicians have a mission to help patients achieve lasting change. Even though people may exhibit similar symptoms and common complaints, physicians are called upon to recognize each individual's unique perspective and treat accordingly. I know that for myself and my colleagues, caring for patients means *caring* above all else—without compromise of quality and without personal agendas. We each accepted in all sincerity the universal oath that is the *sine qua non* of medical practice: Do no harm.

Appreciative Dialogue is more than a "health care program." It is a fundamental shift in the way we view our lives, one that fully embraces a vision of goodness. With this revolutionary method, we achieve a reflective yet powerfully interactive concept of healing. Whether patient or colleague, we share a common bond to recognize and fulfill our dreams.

Appreciative

Feeling grateful or
thankful for.
Being fully aware
or conscious of.
Valuing.

Dialogue

Exchange of conversation, ideas,
or agreement between two or
more people.
To discuss areas of uncertainty
frankly in order to resolve them.

A Workbook for
Your Healing Journey
Using Appreciative Dialogue

It may appear that we are a reflection of our world—
our own experiences, our environment, our relationships.
However, our true inner self is the reflection of our soul,
the spirit that makes us unique.
To access this is nothing short of a miracle.

*T*here are only two ways to live your life.
One is as though nothing is a miracle.
The other is as though everything is a miracle.

~ ALBERT EINSTEIN

The foundation of
this book is the
interconnectedness
of us all—the
thread that spins
a web that truly
connects our lives.

CREATING A HEALTH CARE ALTERNATIVE

As a medical student, I cherished the opportunity to study the art of medicine. Like countless others, I was motivated by a desire to help people and to assist in alleviating pain and suffering. I deeply wished to make a difference—and to make my own life meaningful. However, I was astounded at how little healing was actually being accomplished. In medical school, role models were few, and the uncaring attitude of some specialists toward patients was shocking. I did my residency in Family Practice, perhaps the most humane area of modern medicine, but I still found treatment options and modalities limited—and limiting.

Granted, the medical model has revolutionized the quality of our lives. As we enter a new millennium, we see the incredible advances brought about by technology. But, despite great breakthroughs, many people feel abandoned by conventional medicine. When someone is diagnosed with a disease pattern—such as chronic fatigue syndrome or low back pain—this person inevitably faces a sea of x-rays, lab tests, referrals, and consultations.

As I listened to my patients, however, I discovered a whole new realm of treatment options not considered as viable in my world of university medical centers. These "alternative" modalities consisted mostly of hands-on, non-invasive techniques and benign remedies seldom in conflict with conventional medicine. Nevertheless, they were at odds with its *practitioners*.

1.

Is Complementary Medicine an Alternative?

A new avenue was desperately needed. Everywhere, I encountered patient dissatisfaction, problem patching, fragmentation of therapies, skyrocketing costs, and compromised services within the managed care system. Meanwhile, what we call alternative or complementary medicine had exploded into a 27-billion-dollar industry—a figure comparable to the combined out-of-pocket expenditures of all U.S. physician services.[1] Still, patients were left without a true alternative. That is, these treatment options merely perpetuated the same limited *problem-oriented* approach.

Nonetheless, people were flocking to unconventional types of health care, with or without a physician's blessing. Why? I needed to educate myself beyond what I had learned in medical school. So I began reading books, attending seminars, and conversing with naturopaths, chiropractors, and acupuncturists about a more *holistic* possibility. But, after many impressive presentations from the best within the alternative movement, I had yet to hear anything truly alternative.

What would it take to provide patients with a healing experience that included self-design, choice, collaboration, and optimum solutions? I felt compelled to create and implement such an *integrative* system, realizing it would require an overall paradigm shift in consciousness.

The term "alternative medicine" is used to refer to modalities of healing that are not taught in conventional (allopathic) medical schools. As alternative medicine becomes more accepted, the new trend is to address these modalities as "complementary." These terms are used interchangeably in this book. Additionally, as various treatment regimes merge, this may be referred to as an *integrative approach*.

How Will a Paradigm Shift Foster Healing?

A paradigm refers to the way we see the world or, more specifically, how our mind sees the world. We continuously interpret the stimuli we are exposed to and filter them through the cells of our central nervous system.

Our response to the outer world usually depends upon previous experiences and conditioning—our programming. We might not realize that we are already set up to respond in a given way. For example, do you recognize when you are reacting against your own best interests? We often excuse this kind of subjective self-sabotage as human nature. More accurately, it is a limiting way of using our mind.

If problems and crises dominate daily life, then we may habitually view our experience from a negative paradigm. And, if we focus on these problems, we may never get beyond complaints. The exciting prospect is that we *can* change our perspective. In fact, we can change our entire inner chemistry—the biological reactions of our physiology.

In a cascading effect, human physiology results from chemical reactions which affect and are affected by emotions. By changing our emotional state and our mindset, we have a better possibility of healing. Hence, a positive outlook is a necessary prelude to "feeling great."

What Is Integrative Medicine?

I thought there must be a way for individuals to create the positive emotional states required for maximum healing. As a physician, I knew that there should also be a way for practitioners to work together in order to understand their patients' needs.

My focus changed rapidly to an emerging idea. Why not bridge the diverse segments of health care and patient needs with an interactive communication system? Wouldn't this create a synergy among a wide array of professionals while optimizing personal well-being?

I tackled the parameters of an integrative dialogue for wellness and devised *Appreciative Dialogue*, which lets health care professionals know what is really going on with their patients. Specifically, this process explores and exposes the perceptions patients have of themselves. *Appreciative Dialogue* will forge relationships between practitioners of both complementary and conventional medicine and create integrative protocols. By means of a journal and unifying protocols, communication is enhanced across disciplines and amongst various types of people and situations. What is the method's noteworthy contribution? It takes advantage of each individual's unique *positive* attributes. Thus, *Appreciative Dialogue* asks probing questions, clarifying an individual's choices by eliciting the ideal—his or her hopes and dreams.

Miracles happen when patients self-design their own guides through medicine's maze of physicians, therapists, and allied health professionals. At the same time, practitioners begin to revitalize their interactions with patients, transforming themselves as well. Indeed, *Appreciative Dialogue* assists all of us to find the correct balance. If complementary medicine is to flourish and continue to grow, we need to view diverse modalities from an alternative paradigm—an integrative approach that will span the continuum of health care.

1. D. M. Eisenberg, R. B. Davis, S. L. Ettner, S. Appel, S. Wilkey, M. Van Rompay, R. C. Kessler. 1998. "Trends in Alternative Medicine Use in the United States, 1980-1997." *Journal of American Medical Association,* 280, 1569-1575.

I connect with
all living things
by first being
one with myself.

WHAT IS *APPRECIATIVE DIALOGUE* ?

I have prepared this book to aid your healing process. In itself, it is a therapeutic modality meant to release a wealth of new ideas. By completing the workbook pages that follow, you will have answered questions about your own requirements for health and fulfillment. These, in turn, will help create a new reality of infinite possibilities.

I invite you to open a dialogue with your innermost fears and desires, drawing on all of your personal experience. Then, share this journal with health care providers in order to gain rapport and knowledge. As professionals begin to assist you, they can optimize a plan that is uniquely yours. The vital partnerships you form as a result will increase your ability to achieve total wellness.

Appreciative Dialogue in a Nutshell

Seven points summarize the vision of *Appreciative Dialogue*:

1. An individualized, proactive, patient-centered approach to holistic solutions for health and healing.
2. An interactive format of self-discovery for patients with any chronic (not acute) medical condition (such as fibromyalgia, depression, and chronic pain syndrome).
3. A way to redirect personal focus, thus tapping the ability to harness innate healing energetics within each individual's own immune system.
4. A protocol for generating choices for those who want to view life positively, consider infinite possibilities, and foster optimal health.

5. A plan that encourages mutual, synergistic relationships between empowered patients and a full range of practitioners in an environment of recognition and respect.
6. An opportunity for health care practitioners to recapture their enthusiasm for the practice of medicine.
7. A vehicle to create integrative health care, whereby complementary networks of healing will flourish in communities across the nation.

Who Benefits Most From Appreciative Dialogue?

Appreciative Dialogue brings forth an emotional state that allows for maximum healing. It helps to release endogenous physiological reactions and catalyze innate healing systems. For example, when you call upon past experiences of joy, laughter, and exhilaration, in any given moment you can harness all that is necessary to address a challenging situation.

Yet, no matter how wonderful this system, your conscious mind needs to acknowledge that *choices are possible.* It is not enough to generate solutions and mark out a creative strategy. To truly experience lasting change, you must first set the stage—by making a *commitment to the process.* Your intent thus commands a positive mindset, in which healing options can proliferate.

This is not a quick answer to the complex issues of life. **It will take time and require your active participation in journal writings and partnering with a health care professional.** As a journey of life, *Appreciative Dialogue* demands an investment of your energy in order for you to reach the peak of health and fitness.

The challenge is simply to begin. You must be still and evoke the courage. Listen inwardly. Embrace your internal feelings, emotions, and aspirations. As you start to see the world anew, your entire body chemistry will respond. This is not just "positive thinking," but a new way of life that transforms heartfelt dreams and powerful solutions into daily experience.

What Makes This Method Different?

First, *Appreciative Dialogue* recognizes only solutions. In contrast, most practitioners adopt a problem-oriented format, such as

*   How can I help you?
*   What seems to be the problem?
*   What brings you in today?

In fact, when physicians admit patients to the hospital, a typical sequence is the following:

- The chief complaint is . . .
- The patient presented complaining of . . .
- The history of the presenting illness is . . .

These may be valid questions and statements, but do they offer positive, creative strategies from which to view solutions? For medicine to be truly integrative, there must be a complete restructuring of the physician-patient encounter.

In *Appreciative Dialogue,* the initial interview process is actually therapeutic. Patient "problems" are reframed from an individual perspective, unleashing an unmistakable response from within—a healing force that begs to be called forth. This opens up a truly alternative paradigm.

Second, this system respects cultural, religious, and ethnic diversity. At first glance, the interactive approach may appear somewhat abstract. However, it establishes a practical way to discuss concepts such as your "soul" and "spirit" with professionals in the context of healing.

I believe that unless we understand our inner self, it may be difficult to achieve the miracles we know are possible. Only by recognizing our uniqueness, by embracing our spirituality, can we develop our entire being to experience those miracles.

This book, however, is not about religion. It should not offend any belief system. Nor does it advocate a particular perspective, although prayer is an extremely powerful force. Foremost, this is a celebration of a multitude of pathways . . . and an opportunity to find peace and harmony within.

Is This Preventative Medicine?

The cry can be heard . . . from the corner delicatessen to the corridors of our great medical institutions. We are demanding more basic, more "natural" avenues to healing. We want therapies that are less invasive, more holistic. We are seeking a voice and asking for control over our destiny.

Practitioners are learning to value *Appreciative Dialogue*—a simple, intuitive, easily accessed look into patients' concerns and overall health. This is preventative medicine in its purest state, the beginning of conscious, directed health care. Most importantly, you will play an *active* role, along with a unified team of professionals determined to reach your special goals.

You are a pioneer of healing along with many others. Together we will keep listening to our hearts and nourishing our souls. At the helm of our personal journey, we are spreading a wellness concept that will surely reverberate across the country. This intent for the unification of complementary and conventional health choices will change the face of medicine forever.

As more people experience optimal health—made accessible by direction and connection—we also will witness a growing network of healing practitioners. In truth, a dynamic organization of servers—from cardiologists to chiropractors, family physicians to Ayurvedic practitioners—will be welcomed by all providers who think holistically. Hence, working with this individualized format we will systematically and cohesively begin to manifest collective rewards. Today brings hope and a helping hand as we travel together toward dreams yet to be realized.

 I create synergistic relationships with all that is positive. This allows me to experience a giant leap ahead toward infinite possibilities.

APPRECIATIVE DIALOGUE AT WORK

We all face challenges in life. They are part of our journey. And each journey is a story, usually not that much different from our own.

Throughout this book, you will encounter composite case studies from my practice reflecting aspects of *Appreciative Dialogue* in action. These represent a variety of insights gleaned over the past few years in working with the individual challenges of several patients. I hope that these patient stories will help inspire your next step. You will find a more detailed and personal account, Jonathan's Story, in the following pages. In addition, I have included excerpts from my own healing journey in Sections A through D.

Please note that references to chemotherapy or other invasive treatment should not be taken as contrary to the protocol of *Appreciative Dialogue*. Such measures may of necessity be an ingredient in someone's treatment plan. This book is primarily about finding your own unique path to wellness. Therefore, your process is specific to you and should contain no predetermined elements or outcomes.

Jonathan's Story

Basically, I've had everything I could ask for in life.

I've always been very optimistic about the world and my role in it; I've had a good life. But one day, I found a lump under my right arm.

A month after feeling that lump, I found myself in the office of Dr. Roy. It was then that I learned what an oncologist was and what a biopsy meant. After the initial shock of discovering that the lump was malignant (that is, cancer), I knew I would do everything in my power to beat it. I wanted not just to survive, but to triumph over a circumstance that appeared to be spiraling out of control.

I began to feel my life was over. I felt a loss of control over my very existence. I couldn't sleep, I couldn't think. Cancer, my disease, consumed my whole life with fear, including my entire thought process. Moreover, I was overwhelmed by opinions about what I should do. It was all very confusing. I needed a plan to regain my sense of optimism and to know I could win over this invasion of my body.

It was at that time I learned about *Appreciative Dialogue*. I remember it was another perfect day in the idyllic town of Pacific Grove when I first met Tel Franklin. We were at a small patio diner—a spot with fresh delicacies from the Monterey Bay—where everyone smiles and knows your first name. As we talked, I shared with Dr. Franklin that I was in the midst of a battle—the fight of and for my life. He offered to work with me in a unique approach to healing, which he called *Appreciative Dialogue*, a new way for patients and doctors to envision optimal health. (Note to the reader: Jonathan was not residing in California–so being his physician was not an option at that time.)

Here I share the greatest story of my life, and perhaps the most challenging path for "all" human beings—the healing journey of self-discovery. Initially, I had talked with friends and family about my needs. It became clear that I needed to partner with a primary care physician who would be my guide (one of the first steps of the *Appreciative Dialogue* process).

I must have interviewed thirty doctors before I met Dr. Clay. I felt one hundred percent comfortable with him. He spoke softly and was not rushed. He agreed to meet with me every ten days to review my progress and journal writing. He truly saw my struggle as *our* struggle, and I used our good rapport as a benchmark for screening all other practitioners.

One of my biggest challenges was finding practitioners who would partner with me. I interviewed just short of eighty professionals. Of these, I saw five on a regular schedule and am continuing with three now. Those doctors who would not consent to an initial screening session were omitted from consideration. Nonetheless, most physicians consented to a five-minute consultation without charge. A good approach is to send a letter of introduction explaining your intention (see Addendum A).

As I look back to this period, I am literally amazed at the networking and how one practitioner would suggest another and then another, all working with me—adopting the *Appreciative Dialogue* methods I had learned.

My primary care doctor, Dr. Clay, was an angel sent from heaven, diligently researching and connecting me with those who would later be my partners. And it was those professionals who continued to guide me. Although I chose some and not others, everyone was supportive. I really built my own healing network, practitioner by practitioner.

Without exception, *Appreciative Dialogue* inspired me to "expect a miracle." Its structure gave me the right blend of insight and focus for the path ahead, for I began my journey envisioning a positive outcome.

Like most patients, my initial encounters took the course of conventional (allopathic) medicine. Even though most of the physicians were supportive and kind, they were reluctant to depart from their usual protocols. They acknowledged complementary therapies, but often lacked an understanding of how best to apply them.

After the removal of the tumor, I elected to continue with routine follow-up (lab tests and examinations) but declined any additional invasive treatment (such as chemotherapy). My oncologist was very supportive. Instead, I began to critique each modality that I saw as a potential option using the *Appreciative Dialogue* format. This was a critical element in determining the most meaningful treatment options. I reviewed each modality, writing down my expectations before starting the treatment. The final outcomes often differed, but setting the tone and detailing my expectations was essential to the process. Almost immediately after participating in a particular modality, I would write down my perceived benefits at various time intervals: immediately after treatment and again six, twenty-four, and forty-eight hours later. I also rated the modalities compared to my expectations before beginning treatment (see Addendum B).

The journal writings of *Appreciative Dialogue* included a conversation with myself. This personal reflection helped clarify where I was on my path and where my journey needed to take me. It was this inner vision that gave me balance and direction throughout my adventure.

I always felt calmer and more at peace after spending twenty to forty minutes just writing. It was a kind of catharsis not unlike unloading with your best friend: no judgment, only unconditional acceptance and support. My journal helped me understand my inner self a little better.

Using a process of visualization, I could almost see my day before I even got out of bed each morning. I would spend quiet time (about five to ten minutes) creating the day I wanted. I knew without a doubt that my body was dependent upon *me* to heal. This was an enormous source of strength, and it fueled my determination to be at my best, to *Expect a Miracle* each day.

This changed my life and opened a whole new world full of possibilities. Through the questions and answers of *Appreciative Dialogue,* I discovered ME. I am more aware of how I am feeling and what those emotions mean. Most of all, this growing sensitivity allows me to creatively use my instinct to optimize any situation.

Another essential ingredient to healing has been my family—my parents and siblings, and also relatives I had not talked to or heard from in years. They call, write, or e-mail with the love and support that truly lifts my spirit. These are folks with whom I had grown up and who know my roots. This has proven itself to be real unconditional love, essential for healing.

I find the integration of acupuncture, chiropractic, and massage a tremendous help. The time I make to walk barefoot on the beach is golden. I awaken at least once a week at 5:00 a.m. to watch the sunrise. I never go to sleep mad and am always truthful and honest. I do nothing that is not in my best interest. I have indeed discovered who my friends are. I have learned to be selfish, to care about others, to listen to my body, to thoroughly enjoy the day, to fully share life with others, and to appreciate the precious gift of giving.

I also enjoy sharing my journey with friends, acquaintances, and fellow patients I've met through support groups. The expression "You can't do it alone" has special meaning for me. Even now, I continue to tell my story so that others may glimpse their own potential journey.

In addition to working at a job that I love, I try to make the atmosphere healthy for others. I spend thirty minutes a day in quiet meditation. I take some time to sit by the ocean. Except for Sundays, I run or walk at least thirty minutes daily. I now regularly shop at the open-air farmer's market. I eat only organically grown foods—small servings, but six meals a day. I tell my mom and dad "I love you" before hanging up the phone. There are some "friends" I don't see anymore. I also screen my phone calls and am selective about whom I call back. I volunteer to give my young niece and nephew a bath, or just spend time with them and do what they choose. I make it a point not to rush— especially while driving. And I don't say "hate" anymore. I remember all the things I love, and I enjoy those moments over and over again. I still see a chiropractor every eight weeks and have energetic acupuncture every twelve weeks.

It has been two years since the original diagnosis of cancer, and there is no trace of a tumor. I have reached a peak of life. My journey has taken me from the depths of despair to a height that has redefined the meaning of my existence. I am not the only one who has grown. Most of the practitioners I have worked with, including Dr. Clay, my primary care physician, now share how they have gone from only limited knowledge of *Appreciative Dialogue* to professional and personal lives that have been forever changed.

Today, I live each moment as a gift. I know that in any given situation there are choices, and I accept full responsibility for my decisions. *Appreciative Dialogue* is the way I view life and the way I live it every day. I know the old paradigm is still there, but with the excitement and thrill of today, I'll never go back. There will always be obstacles and criticism from certain friends, but I can see past any negativity or challenges and enjoy overcoming all barriers to live the miracle of life today.

The most important lessons I've learned are to hold a universal love for all living beings, to continuously suspend judgment, and to always live in the moment—only then will miracles be the norm. My life has been fully transformed.

J.S.S.

 Without limitations,
every moment is a miracle.

I acknowledge
the day and
embrace it with
the energy of life.

TO BEGIN THE HEALING JOURNEY

Expect a Miracle is an interactive guide that can be used for exploring and accessing a broad range of therapeutic healing modalities. Sections A through D involve the need for deep personal reflection and require your written responses to questions. Your journal will prove most beneficial if revisited on a continuing basis, especially after periods of in-depth reevaluation. Remember, you are the most powerful witness to your own healing journey.

The chapters ahead guide you through four distinct yet synergistic processes using *Appreciative Dialogue.* Be prepared for the self-dialogue to release strong emotional energies. For most people, this natural healing response makes way for a peaceful flow of increasing awareness and transformation.

However, all journal writing (after Section A's ten questions) **should be undertaken with the support and guidance of your physician.** Sharing your journey with a health care professional leads to a second kind of interactive dialogue, giving you the greatest opportunity to actualize your desires and dreams.

The four steps that will constitute your individual script for health are:

Section A. First Steps to Self-Awareness
Section B. Modalities That Nurture
Section C. Keys to New Directions
Section D. Actualization of the Ultimate Self

A. First Steps to Self-Awareness

When setting out on a journey, the first thing to do is look at a map. Your written responses in Section A will define the "geography" of your health. With this self-awareness you can create a visual image of where you are at this time. Just as an explorer prepares to scale mountainous heights from the vantage point of base camp, you will begin with a pre-journey reference point of who you are right now—in body, mind, and spirit. From the clarity of your inner reflection, you will ultimately build a unique plan for future travels to the destination of well-being.

B. Modalities That Nurture

Understanding the possible therapies in Section B is a conscious step into the domain of health care choices. In the same way that an adventurer takes stock of various resources to reach a particular goal, you too will look for multiple vehicles to reach optimal health. For example, the adventurer might travel by horseback and trek on foot through a mountain wilderness after taking a jeep to get to the Sierras. Likewise, you might call upon the "vehicles" of exercise and vitamin supplements after a course of chiropractic adjustments.

The idea is to gain access to the best of both complementary and conventional modalities. "Best" is determined by your specific needs and desires as facilitated by your health care provider. By way of this partnering, an integrative, personalized protocol can be implemented that will help you meet and even surpass your goals.

C. Keys to New Directions

Your responses in Section C point to the destinations you most wish to explore. When you look at a map of the world, you may be tempted to visit many places. In order to reach Zanzibar, Bhutan, and the Loire Valley, however, a plan is essential. Your answers here provide a key to the new directions you will actually follow. Next, you will be able to create a plan for your life and focus on where you are going. This is the way to quantify your progress and consciously exceed all expectations.

D. Actualization of the Ultimate Self

Completing the statements in Section D allows you to draw on the power of your achievements. You will be able to recognize, appreciate, and access a lasting image of wellness.

When standing at the top of the mountain or cooling down after your best run, there is a moment of body-soul perfection and unification. But physical activity is only one way to achieve this state of actualization. Perhaps the "green flash" of the setting sun, your child's smile at the end of the day, or a glimpse of a humpback whale during migration will also stimulate a physiological change in your body's chemistry, after which a euphoria permeates your being. Such exaltation can unlock the treasures of the universe—to let you become all that you desire.

After completing these four processes, there is a final opportunity to bring together all that you have explored. This summarizing section, called the Optimal Health Plan, will be explained later, after you have experienced more of *Appreciative Dialogue*. First is a step-by-step plan for getting the most out of your Healing Journey.

I challenge myself by embarking on the ultimate voyage . . .
the healing journey of self-discovery.

APPRECIATIVE DIALOGUE STEP-BY-STEP

1. **Read** the entire book. Although you may find some sections beyond your current grasp, it is important to read the entire book, possibly more than once.

2. **Answer** the ten questions in Section A: First Steps to Self-Awareness (pp. 23–36).

3. **Seek out** a physician or health care professional who is willing to explore various modalities and treatment options and who is able to assist you in developing an Optimal Health Plan.

4. **Critique** each treatment you *choose* to experience in Section B: Modalities That Nurture (pp. 39–87), listing that treatment's positive attributes. Note any questions you wish to share with your health practitioner(s). Feel free to critique any additional therapeutic options that are not listed, using the same question-response format.

5. **Assess** your progress in your journal by answering the questions in Section C: Keys to New Directions and Section D: Actualization of the Ultimate Self (see pp. 91 and 107, respectively).

6. **Summarize** your plan of action using the format in the Optimal Health Plan. Do this in conjunction with your physician (see p. 123).

7. **Continue** to review your journal entries with your health care provider. Discuss your questions and share reflections concerning your treatment options.

8. **Share** your journey with those close to you.

9. **Re-read** the entire book. Continue to review and add to your journal writings. Reflect on your growth and discovery of your inner strength and overall health.

10. **Witness** how a cognitive change in your thinking has *transformed* your life.

In responding to the questions, remember the answers are uniquely yours— not right or wrong, only yours.

A Journal of Self-Discovery

The greatest discovery of any generation
is that human beings can alter their lives
by altering the attitudes of their minds.
~ ALBERT SCHWEITZER

*F*ill your journal with the experience
of "Life." Set aside time to write in
A Healing Journey of Self-Discovery.
Try not to discard any pages—all your
thoughts and feelings have validity.
Just begin to express yourself without
regard to grammar or structure. The
questions will access an energetic
system of healing that will begin to
open a dialogue.

Section A: First Steps to Self-Awareness

Appreciative Dialogue reframes the idea of you as a "patient." From now on, you will look at health care practitioners as resources to assist you through a journey of self-discovery. No longer relegated to two-minute prescription refills or constant referrals, you will actively help to direct the course of your treatment.

Throughout the following pages, you will peer into your individuality—an invaluable tool in the quest for optimal health. You possess a powerful spirit that gives meaning to your existence beyond the imprint of your DNA. This ability to realize your most intimate dreams is the true reason for life.

This is neither a new technology nor a search for a mystic power. It is a silent journey in which you will transform yourself to experience the best that is possible. Acting as a guide, *Appreciative Dialogue* asks these questions: What has brought you to this place? How can you help yourself? What is uniquely you? *The time has come to cast away how others have previously defined you.*

At this moment, focus on the positive realm of goodness and health within you. Strength comes from recognizing this vital force. Then, proceed to the questions that follow, an exercise to stimulate the patterns of your energetic healing system.

I encourage you to set aside time each day to celebrate what makes you special. Go inward so you can appreciate the journey forward. As you define the path ahead, you will open a window to your soul. The questions in Sections A through D are first listed, then adequate space follows to allow for your participation.

1. What are the **major factors** that help me maintain health?
2. What are the **minor factors** that help me maintain health?
3. What do I **do** on a daily, weekly, and monthly basis to enjoy health?
4. What **emotions** will I experience when I achieve an increase in health?
5. What **goals** will I achieve as I enjoy an increase in health?
6. What does **optimal health** mean to me?
7. What are my **images** and **past experiences** of optimal health?
8. What can I **do** on a daily, weekly, and monthly basis to experience optimal health?
9. Right now, how can I achieve total optimal health for **one moment**? How can I extend this time frame?
10. How can I **reinforce** this positive behavior on a daily basis?

Gabrielle's Story

Gabrielle visited my office three and a half years ago. At the age of thirty-four, she felt destined to be alone and had stopped counting the number of her failed relationships. She remarked that no one really understood her, and, when they did, they would leave.

The multiple options approach was especially helpful here, for Gabrielle had a number of unresolved issues. First, she completed the *Healing Journey* questions, really getting to understand herself. She also began participating in bimonthly counseling with a trained psychologist, Dr. Lea. Gabrielle introduced her psychologist to *Expect a Miracle* and *Appreciative Dialogue*. Dr. Lea reviewed Gabrielle's journal entries and became an enthusiastic supporter; together they developed an entire network of practitioners. She has also discovered Reiki and Feldenkrais.

She has begun a support group for people in her community interested in pursuing *Appreciative Dialogue*. In this way, Gabrielle feels she is giving back—which helps reinforce her commitment to always look forward. Additionally, I continue to see Gabrielle every eight weeks to review her *Healing Journey* and discuss her progress.

She meditates daily and has become an amateur triathlete. She takes night classes in massage and is a frequent speaker at community groups and schools. She speaks on communication skills in relationships and trust issues within the family.

One day Gabrielle wrote about her summer visits with her grandparents in upstate New York. She recalled the peaceful feeling of sitting alone. She found the rippling blue waters of the mountain lake almost hypnotic. Today when she meditates, she is able to return to her tranquil memories of her childhood and feel in touch with her natural self.

At the end of one of her recent visits, as she walked out of the office, she gazed back and remarked, "You know, Doc, there are no tomorrows . . . and today is the best it's ever been!"

Nature heals. Each day spend time with the smell of fresh air, the ocean crashing on the shore, the sound of rain, the stillness of the sunset. Make this a priority.

What are the **major factors** that help me maintain health?

Date	Entry

Excerpts from Dr. Tel

9-3-00

1) *I have an optimistic view of life.*

2) *I feel connected—friends, family, work, my community.*

3) *I spend time every day with my loyal friend—my dog Kitt.*

4) *I volunteer often—my time, ideas, money.*

5) *I feel good about who I am becoming as a human being.*

6) *I eat simple, healthy food every day—on Sundays, I splurge.*

7) *I feel the love of my life every time I gaze into Jessica's eyes.*

8) *I surround myself with my favorite art and music every day.*

9) *I say what I feel—without being abrasive or rude.*

10) *I enjoy my life—every day.*

Take the first step in the healing journey of self-discovery.

1. What are the **major factors** that help me maintain health?

Date · Entry

2. What are the **minor factors** that help me maintain health?

Date   Entry

Appreciative Dialogue is a journey to a world of possibilities.

3. What do I **do** on a daily, weekly, and monthly basis to enjoy health?

Date · *Entry*

4.   What **emotions** will I experience when I achieve an increase in health?

Date   Entry

Appreciative Dialogue seeks and recognizes your vital living force.

5. What **goals** will I achieve when I enjoy an increase in health?

Date · *Entry*

6. What does **optimal health** mean to me?

Date   Entry

All participants will be forever changed.

7. What are my **images** and **past experiences** of optimal health?

Date   *Entry*

8. What can I **do** on a daily, weekly, and monthly basis to experience optimal health?

Date · *Entry*

Conceptual thought brings forth new ideas . . .

9. Right now, how can I achieve total optimal health for **one moment**?
   How can I extend this time frame?

Date · Entry

10. How can I **reinforce** this positive behavior on a daily basis?

Date	Entry

A paradigm shift spurs the birth of a new society.

Reflection

Begin in silence. Quiet the mind.

Witness the breath. Believe in yourself.

Listen to your heart, spirit, and soul.

By experiencing yourself, you release

a potential energetic force

to create miracles and beyond.

Live each day with heart,

and nothing is left to chance.

You will be amazed by the fulfillment

at day's end.

If I were to wish for anything,

I should not wish for wealth and power,

but for the passionate sense of the potential,

for the vision which, ever young and ardent,

sees the possible.

~ KIERKEGAARD

Section B: Modalities That Nurture

This second stage of your Healing Journey is about *taking inventory.* You will be asked to comment on each option that you have experienced, or would like to experience. It is a lot easier to get to your destination if you know where you have been. Never mind that the roads already traveled for some have been many and for others few.

Consider the following modalities as resources for tapping into a vital energy force that can create healing and more. Many choices reflect a holistic approach, recognizing the connection of mind, body, and soul. I have found that most people respond well to a full spectrum of modalities. It is the application of the right combinations at optimal times and intervals that releases maximum healing potential.

The following list is not meant to be definitive. Countless fine therapies have not been included. For example, the planet's indigenous cultures have long benefited from valid health alternatives—some since the beginning of civilization. On the other hand, if certain treatment options appear strange or unfamiliar, just move on. Or undertake in-depth research for a better understanding. There is ample space to explore whatever ideas you would like to try, so add any modalities that interest you.

It is important to evaluate your choices with critical thinking. To accomplish that, I advise you to learn the basics of statistical analysis. Further, ask professionals for scientific data to support an informed decision. Learn what results are expected and consider the most likely outcomes. By the way, your physician may be an excellent resource in the evaluation of such data.

Also, note that "natural" does not necessarily mean healthier or better for *you.* Many naturally occurring substances are toxic. And most pharmaceuticals have known side effects. Please look to your physician in order to minimize harmful effects of all medicines, herbs, or botanicals.

For cancer patients, allopathic (conventional medicine) protocols may include chemotherapy, radiation treatments, bone marrow transplants, or stem cell therapy as part of a viable, life-saving plan. It is important to discuss all options with your physician. You can ask how to mitigate any adverse side effects that may arise.

I experience optimal health by gaining access to vital energetic systems.

It has been my good fortune to witness the decision-making processes of my patients as they struggle for the best choices. Fulfillment comes when we ask the right questions and then listen to our heart. The knowledge we gain from *Appreciative Dialogue* opens doors that previously appeared impassable.

Modalities

Think of the following treatment options as tools for harnessing a vital energetic force that can create a synergistic healing system. Each modality you choose is a resource to release the inner healing spirit—a life force that all human beings possess. In the following pages, each modality is briefly defined.

1. Conventional-Allopathic Medicine
2. Traditional Chinese Medicine / Acupuncture
3. Aromatherapy
4. Ayurveda
5. Chiropractic
6. Exercise
7. Feldenkrais / Somatics
8. Functional Medicine
9. Herbs / Botanicals
10. Homeopathy
11. Hypnosis
12. Guided Imagery / Visualization
13. Massage
14. Naturopathy
15. Nutrition
16. Osteopathic Medicine
17. Reiki / Therapeutic Touch / Energy Force
18. Rolfing / Structural Integration
19. Spirituality
20. Vitamin and Mineral Supplementation
21. Yoga / Qi Gong / Tai Chi

Joseph's Story

Joseph is a 63-year-old mechanic who developed back pain after manually lifting a transmission—the electric hoist had broken earlier in the week.

Besieged by coaxing from co-workers, Joseph consented to see Dr. Elm, a local chiropractor. Following a brief exam, the chiropractor promptly called the paramedics and Joseph was taken to the local emergency room. He was diagnosed with an aortic aneurysm and scheduled for immediate surgery.

Shortly after his rehabilitation, Joseph arranged a consultation with my office. He confessed that he had almost always suppressed his emotions, especially if feeling sad or depressed. "I guess I wasn't ever taught to really express myself," Joseph shared. "You were supposed to just deal with it."

Joseph has since participated in *Appreciative Dialogue,* helping him to rethink his priorities. He now appreciates the life he once took for granted. He continually comments on how *Appreciative Dialogue* has transformed his life. "I'm no longer afraid to say how I feel, and I'm able to listen to others when they share with me." Joseph spends almost thirty minutes every night just reflecting on the day and joyfully contemplating tomorrow.

Joseph has lost almost 110 pounds—and is now down to 185. His cholesterol ratios have improved by greater than 250%. He enjoys daily sunrise walks with his wife. Although two years ago he had never heard the word "vegan," now he's "as strict as they come." New cholesterol-lowering medications, along with his amazing lifestyle changes, have significantly added quality as well as years to his life. He makes regular "dates" with his grandchildren and has planned his first trip to the Grand Canyon. He plans to walk the entire rim with his eldest daughter.

That fateful day which almost took Joseph away has changed him into a man who supremely enjoys the breath of life. His priority is now to celebrate every day for what it is: a precious gift.

I am taking advantage of all opportunities to smile, laugh, and just have fun!

Excerpts from Dr. Tel

MASSAGE

Massage is the manipulation of soft tissue for therapeutic purposes, primarily to relieve pain, stiffness, stress, and fatigue. Varied approaches involve different techniques, but in general massage therapy increases circulation and lymph flow, delivery of oxygen and nutrients to muscle tissue, and removal of metabolic waste and other toxic substances from the body.

—How I define it:

The act of "therapeutic touch"—a special time for myself.

—My personal experience:

Almost always feel more relaxed, especially throughout the next week— an essential ingredient to feeling good.

—Positive feeling associated with it:

I feel more conscious about my muscles and the ability to just be still and feel my body move freely.

In this moment I acknowledge the character
of my soul—the essence of my being.

—What I feel it may offer:

Helps to keep me flexible and elevates my feelings of well-being.

Also, decreases tension in muscles and allows me to enjoy

movement more.

—Desired outcome—my objective:

To continually increase my sense of well-being and

minimize stress/strain on joints. To allow relaxation to

permeate my entire body.

—Feel free to make any other comments or share any thoughts:

Date · *Entry*

9-13-00 · *An essential ingredient to maintaining optimal health and*

· *well-being. A cornerstone in my regimen of overall fitness*

· *and prevention of imbalances.*

1. CONVENTIONAL-ALLOPATHIC MEDICINE

Allopathic medicine refers to conventional Western health care. Allopathy relies on pharmaceuticals, surgery, and areas of specialization. Practitioners may include your family physician and specialists such as a cardiologist, ophthalmologist, psychologist, podiatrist, or other trained, licensed health care professionals.

—How I define it:

—My personal experience:

—Positive feeling associated with it:

—What I feel it may offer:

—Desired outcome—my objective:

—Feel free to make any other comments or share any thoughts:

Date	Entry

2. TRADITIONAL CHINESE MEDICINE / ACUPUNCTURE

Traditional Chinese Medicine treats overall health by stimulating specific points in the body by the insertion of needles. The goal is to establish or restore the natural flow of the vital life force (Qi) through energy channels in the body. Please note that acupuncture is but one aspect of TCM. Within this treatment, acupuncture is often combined with herbal remedies for a comprehensive approach. Acupuncture treats a range of conditions including pain, arthritis, addiction, PMS, high blood pressure, and asthma.

—How I define it:

—My personal experience:

—Positive feeling associated with it:

—What I feel it may offer:

_____

_____

_____

_____

_____

—Desired outcome—my objective:

_____

_____

_____

_____

_____

_____

_____

_____

—Feel free to make any other comments or share any thoughts:

Date	Entry

3. AROMATHERAPY

This is the therapeutic use of essential oils extracted from flowers, leaves, roots, or fruits of plants and trees. By inhalation or absorption through the skin, and through bath oils, salts, or diffusers, the oils aid in relieving such complaints as muscle aches, arthritis, and inflammation. They also help to energize, center, or release emotional stress.

—How I define it:

—My personal experience:

—Positive feeling associated with it:

—What I feel it may offer:

_____

_____

_____

_____

_____

—Desired outcome—my objective:

_____

_____

_____

_____

_____

_____

_____

—Feel free to make any other comments or share any thoughts:

Date   *Entry*

4. AYURVEDA

This ancient art and science of healing from India is a preventive and holistic approach that focuses on natural healing through inner harmony. Ayurveda recognizes that basic elements (ether, air, fire, water, and earth) condense in the body and must be balanced for good health. Treatment may be constitutional (diet, herbs, and lifestyle adjustments) or clinical (cleansing and purification).

—How I define it:

—My personal experience:

—Positive feeling associated with it:

—What I feel it may offer:

—Desired outcome—my objective:

—Feel free to make any other comments or share any thoughts:

Date	Entry

5. CHIROPRACTIC

Chiropractic methods focus on correct alignment of the spine to minimize, correct, and prevent structural disorders. Chiropractors treat back, neck, and leg pain, headaches, numbness, and PMS, for example. They are also often alert to other physical or nutritional deficiencies that might cause chronic health problems.

—How I define it:

—My personal experience:

—Positive feeling associated with it:

—What I feel it may offer:

—Desired outcome—my objective:

—Feel free to make any other comments or share any thoughts:

Date	Entry

6. EXERCISE

Physical exercise is the body in motion against gravity. Popular examples today include walking, cycling, swimming, running, stretching, and dancing. Exercise is for a healthy heart, to strengthen muscles and bones, stimulate the immune system, alleviate anxiety or depression, manage stress, and increase mental clarity.

—How I define it:

—My personal experience:

—Positive feeling associated with it:

—What I feel it may offer:

_____

_____

_____

_____

_____

—Desired outcome—my objective:

_____

_____

_____

_____

_____

_____

_____

_____

—Feel free to make any other comments or share any thoughts:

Date	Entry

7. FELDENKRAIS / SOMATICS

These techniques are part of a larger group of healing methods that focus on personal awareness of habitual body positions and movements. Practitioners can identify and help correct problematic areas that cause discomfort, fatigue, and related emotional conditions. In one-to-one sessions or in classes, you will learn specialized movements to enhance awareness and communication between mind and body.

—How I define it:

—My personal experience:

—Positive feeling associated with it:

—What I feel it may offer:

_____

_____

_____

_____

_____

—Desired outcome—my objective:

_____

_____

_____

_____

_____

_____

_____

_____

—Feel free to make any other comments or share any thoughts:

Date	Entry

8. FUNCTIONAL MEDICINE

Functional medicine is a patient-centered system of health care that identifies and addresses a broad range of factors to reverse disease progression and enhance vitality. It employs assessment and early intervention, incorporating solutions from biochemistry, physiology, psychology, and environmental medicine.

—How I define it:

—My personal experience:

—Positive feeling associated with it:

—What I feel it may offer:

_____

_____

_____

_____

_____

—Desired outcome—my objective:

_____

_____

_____

_____

_____

_____

_____

—Feel free to make any other comments or share any thoughts:

Date	Entry

9. HERBS / BOTANICALS

Many plants have medicinal properties in their seeds, berries, roots, leaves, bark, or flowers. Used for millennia in primary health care, herbs are prepared in a variety of ways: infusions, tinctures, powders, pills, liniments, salves, ointments, and syrups. The guidance of a professional is essential when using herbs for therapeutic purposes.

—How I define it:

—My personal experience:

—Positive feeling associated with it:

—What I feel it may offer:

_____

_____

_____

_____

_____

—Desired outcome—my objective:

_____

_____

_____

_____

_____

_____

_____

—Feel free to make any other comments or share any thoughts:

Date	Entry

10. HOMEOPATHY

Homeopathy proceeds under the notion that "like cures like." It views disease as the result of a deep systemic disturbance or imbalance, of which the symptoms are only an outward manifestation. It uses minimum doses of specially prepared plants and minerals to stimulate the body's self-healing mechanisms. Treatment is individualized, taking into consideration the patient's entire physical system, history, lifestyle, and personality.

—How I define it:

—My personal experience:

—Positive feeling associated with it:

—What I feel it may offer:

_____

_____

_____

_____

_____

—Desired outcome—my objective:

_____

_____

_____

_____

_____

_____

_____

_____

—Feel free to make any other comments or share any thoughts:

Date	Entry

11. HYPNOSIS

The goal of hypnosis is to identify and change certain learned behaviors, replacing them with more positive attributes. It acknowledges the influence of the subconscious mind on the body and emotions. Hypnosis is often used along with other therapies to stop smoking, lose weight, manage pain, and ease childbirth.

—How I define it:

—My personal experience:

—Positive feeling associated with it:

—What I feel it may offer:

_____

_____

_____

_____

—Desired outcome—my objective:

_____

_____

_____

_____

_____

_____

_____

—Feel free to make any other comments or share any thoughts:

Date	*Entry*

12. GUIDED IMAGERY / VISUALIZATION

This technique uses a person's mental faculties to deal with pain, control illness, and shape personal goals. In the guided imagery process, a facilitator may help elicit healing images that promote desirable outcomes. Visualization draws on the creative power of the mind to focus on self-generated pictures of health and well-being.

—How I define it:

—My personal experience:

—Positive feeling associated with it:

—What I feel it may offer:

_____

_____

_____

_____

—Desired outcome—my objective:

_____

_____

_____

_____

_____

_____

_____

—Feel free to make any other comments or share any thoughts:

Date	Entry

13. MASSAGE

Massage is the manipulation of soft tissue for therapeutic purposes, primarily to relieve pain, stiffness, stress, and fatigue. Varied approaches involve different techniques, but in general, massage therapy increases circulation and lymph flow, delivery of oxygen and nutrients to muscle tissue, and removal of metabolic waste and other toxic substances from the body.

—How I define it:

—My personal experience:

—Positive feeling associated with it:

—What I feel it may offer:

_____

_____

_____

_____

_____

—Desired outcome—my objective:

_____

_____

_____

_____

_____

_____

_____

_____

—Feel free to make any other comments or share any thoughts:

Date	Entry

14. NATUROPATHY

Naturopathy employs a wide range of alternative therapies in which the patient actively participates. The emphasis is on treatment to support—rather than take over—the body's natural healing processes. The naturopathic approach, which often requires lifestyle changes, seeks not only to alleviate but also to prevent health problems.

—How I define it:

—My personal experience:

—Positive feeling associated with it:

—What I feel it may offer:

—Desired outcome—my objective:

—Feel free to make any other comments or share any thoughts:

Date	Entry

15. NUTRITION

Nutrition as a healing modality involves the assessment of necessary nutrients for corrective or preventive therapy and the following of a diet providing these nutrients. Through a comprehensive regimen, overall health is maintained and disease states may be alleviated. Practitioners can differ greatly in opinion regarding the best type, quantity, and management of ingredients for an ideal diet. Adjunct therapies may include inner cleansing protocols.

—How I define it:

—My personal experience:

—Positive feeling associated with it:

—What I feel it may offer:

_____

_____

_____

_____

_____

—Desired outcome—my objective:

_____

_____

_____

_____

_____

_____

_____

_____

—Feel free to make any other comments or share any thoughts:

Date	Entry

16. OSTEOPATHIC MEDICINE

Osteopathy is a holistic health care system that combines manipulative treatment, similar to chiropractic, with allopathic medicine, nutrition, and exercise. The emphasis is on the interconnectedness of body support systems and a healthy musculo-skeletal system as keys to overall health.

—How I define it:

—My personal experience:

—Positive feeling associated with it:

—What I feel it may offer:

_____
_____
_____
_____
_____

—Desired outcome—my objective:

_____
_____
_____
_____
_____
_____
_____
_____
_____

—Feel free to make any other comments or share any thoughts:

Date	Entry

17. REIKI / THERAPEUTIC TOUCH / ENERGY FORCE

These healing methods use the laying on of hands to stimulate, calm, or balance energy fields in the body. The goal is to correct blocks and imbalances caused by such stressors as physical and emotional problems, anxiety, and pain. Whether a patient has one or many treatments, practitioners seek to maximize relaxation and well-being.

—How I define it:

—My personal experience:

—Positive feeling associated with it:

—What I feel it may offer:

—Desired outcome—my objective:

—Feel free to make any other comments or share any thoughts:

Date	Entry

18. ROLFING / STRUCTURAL INTEGRATION

Rolfing uses intense manipulation of muscle and fascia to restore balance in the body and realign it with the gravitational field. Treatments typically address pain, depleted energy, chronic muscular tension, and the effects of poor posture.

—How I define it:

—My personal experience:

—Positive feeling associated with it:

—What I feel it may offer:

—Desired outcome—my objective:

—Feel free to make any other comments or share any thoughts:

Date	Entry

19. SPIRITUALITY

A spiritual approach to healing acknowledges the power of the mind to influence physiological functions in the body. It also postulates that the individual can control, or at least influence, emotional states and well-being. The spiritual aspect may reflect belief in a higher power to bring healing.

—How I define it:

—My personal experience:

—Positive feeling associated with it:

—What I feel it may offer:

_____

_____

_____

_____

_____

—Desired outcome—my objective:

_____

_____

_____

_____

_____

_____

_____

_____

—Feel free to make any other comments or share any thoughts:

Date	*Entry*

20. VITAMIN AND MINERAL SUPPLEMENTATION

Supplements are taken to ensure the required allowance of certain vitamins and minerals that may not be provided in the daily food intake. Supplements are also recommended to treat specific conditions and correct deficiencies caused by improper diets, strong medications, stressful lifestyles, unhealthy environments, compromised genetics, or underlying medical conditions. Supplementation can come in many forms, from synthetic manufactured isolates to whole, organic plants and foods.

—How I define it:

—My personal experience:

—Positive feeling associated with it:

—What I feel it may offer:

_____

_____

_____

_____

_____

—Desired outcome—my objective:

_____

_____

_____

_____

_____

_____

_____

_____

—Feel free to make any other comments or share any thoughts:

Date	Entry

21. YOGA / QI GONG / TAI CHI

Practicing yoga with its discipline of postures results in increased strength and flexibility, calmness, and overall well-being. Part meditation, part movement, Qi Gong is an ancient Chinese system of healing exercises similar to yoga. It circulates energy and prompts the body toward proper alignment. Tai Chi consists of a series of flowing meditative movements. All of these techniques are centered around clarity, mental focus, and awareness of the breath.

—How I define it:

—My personal experience:

—Positive feeling associated with it:

—What I feel it may offer:

—Desired outcome—my objective:

—Feel free to make any other comments or share any thoughts:

Date	*Entry*

22. OTHER MODALITY

—How I define it:

—My personal experience:

—Positive feeling associated with it:

—What I feel it may offer:

—Desired outcome—my objective:

—Feel free to make any other comments or share any thoughts:

Date · *Entry*

Reflection

We are all interconnected.

There is a universal bond between all people.

When we cease to act as isolated individuals,

we access a spirit that permeates all living beings

and helps us live more fulfilling lives.

It is this synergism that creates miracles.

*B*y focusing on creative strategies
to achieve an optimal healing state,
we change our interaction with and
perception of the universe.

Section C: Keys to New Directions

Through *Appreciative Dialogue,* you have examined a number of complementary modalities, assessed their benefits for your needs, and perhaps tried something new and different. Still, you may not have realized your most deeply-rooted desires.

I invite you to go one step further, rethinking what you have learned on your *Healing Journey.* Ask yourself, "What have I accomplished so far?" This helps clarify your goals and objectives and places you closer to your dreams.

The following questions help you see exactly where you are going and what you aspire to be—they are the key to radiant health. As you answer each one, pay close attention to these three things:

a) Include in your journal the activities and events of joy in your life, the people who make you laugh and smile, and all else that brings happiness to your day. *Cherish what helps you grow and offers peace to your soul.*

b) Bring to your written answers the immediacy of all of your senses—smell, taste, sound, sight, and touch. What will it be like to achieve your soul's desire? Especially remember the power of your thoughts. If you can imagine it, if you can visualize it, *then it is well within your grasp.*

c) Each modality you highlighted in Section B is a potential pathway to vibrant health. Reflect on the totality of your interactions and experiences to *find the unique blend of options best for you.* It is precisely this combination of choices that will propel a quantum leap forward.

Now, focus on your expectations and receive inner guidance. Each time you review the questions, again reassess your journey. For today you have grown, and another horizon is well within reach. Please answer the following questions and/or comment on the statements listed below:

1. What are the subjective and objective criteria I will use to measure my state of well-being? How will I know when I have achieved my goal?

2. What has been the result so far of the modalities I have chosen?

3. How am I closer to my desired outcome of optimal health?

4. What have I learned about my own capacity for healing?

5. How has my perspective or attitude changed?

6. How have I already used an integrative approach in my life? What might I add to this approach in the future?

7. In any situation in which I might feel depleted, I can call upon vital energetic systems that I possess. At any given moment, I may call upon my innate healing energies, such as . . .

8. I will not allow my options to be limited. I *always* have alternatives, and my destiny is shaped by listening to myself—to my heart and soul. Some examples of times that I have *listened* are . . .

9. Optimal health is a dynamic process, the birthright of *all* beings. My optimal self is experienced when I *feel* . . .

10. Optimal health can be expressed only by a unification of mind, body, and spirit. This is to know the soul within. I experience this state when I am . . .

 Appreciative Dialogue is a revolutionary vision of healing and beyond. It challenges our fundamental view of the self within the world at large, introducing a new paradigm of well-being through collaboration and integration.

Genevieve's Story

Genevieve is a very intelligent and articulate 44-year-old woman who came to see me with concerns about her weight. She had once weighed 115 pounds, normal for her 5-foot height and medium build, but now the scale read 211 pounds. "This is the most out of control I have ever been!" she exclaimed. She made little eye contact and even when she did, her tears filled the room with sorrow.

She began with *The Healing Journey* on her initial visit, using *Appreciative Dialogue*. Fifteen months later, Genevieve now awakens early in the morning, has a cup of herbal tea, and enjoys an hour of yoga. She finds that chiropractic adjustments give her vitality and poise. She participates in a weekly women's support group and takes brisk walks daily. Over a period of months, we were able to reduce her anti-depressant medications, so that today she takes no prescription pharmaceuticals. Continuing with her journal, we interact every eight weeks. She has returned to her religious roots and has become a member of an extended interfaith family. She has generated a healing spirit and regained a passion for life. Her journal writing reflects the love and kindness of her new support system and her growing faith.

As long as Genevieve can remember—and perhaps as early as her first step—she had been snow skiing. But nearly twenty years had passed since she stepped into a pair of skis. Recently, Genevieve ventured to the Colorado Rockies on a ski holiday. She could feel her stomach churning as she approached the gondola. After a few runs down the slopes, however, her confidence of childhood was restored. Today, Genevieve recognizes that a return to skiing has given her life focus. As she has challenged herself to traverse steeper mountains and concentrate fully on the terrain ahead, she has also gained the discipline and direction she so desperately needed for her healing journey.

She admits to having more confidence and self-esteem than at any other point in her life. Taking pride in herself, she remarks with joy, "I'm really living. Before, I was just getting by. I realize that life is a gift, and I cherish every precious moment."

The path of my journey is paved with elation. Around every bend I experience a euphoria that can be felt by all.

What are the subjective and objective criteria I will use to determine or measure my state of well-being? How will I know when I've achieved my goal?

Date · Entry

Excerpts from Dr. Tel

9-3-00

1) My energy level throughout the day.

2) How balanced I feel.

3) Mood swings throughout the day.

4) How connected I feel.

5) How I feel at the end of the day—what I was able to accomplish or learn.

6) My clarity of thought.

7) I fall asleep knowing "This day I did my best."

8) There is a synergy of events throughout the day.

9) Feedback from family / friends.

10) After meditating for 30 minutes, I feel as though I am surrounded and protected by an invisible sphere which radiates positive energy and attracts all that I desire.

You are in control of your destiny, directing your life toward the goals that fill you with the spirit of life.

1. What are the subjective and objective criteria I will use to determine or measure my state of well-being? How will I know when I have achieved my goal?

Date · Entry

2.   What has been the result so far of the modalities I have chosen?

Date · *Entry*

Life is not a summation of experiences, rather the expectation of today.

3. How am I closer to my desired outcome of optimal health?

Date *Entry*

4. What have I learned about my own capacity for healing?

Date · *Entry*

When we build self-esteem, we are creating optimal health.
When we understand this, we comprehend that the mind and body are one.

5. How has my perspective or attitude changed?

Date · Entry

The soul is that which makes you a unique human being,
devoid of the ego and as naked as the truth.

6. How have I already used an integrative approach in my life? What might I add
   to this approach in the future?

Date · *Entry*

The spirit is the creative soul which dreams . . .

7. In any situation in which I am feeling depleted, I can call upon vital energetic systems that
    I possess. At any given moment, I may call upon my innate healing energies, such as . . .

Date : *Entry*

8. I will not allow my options to be limited. I *always* have alternatives, and my destiny is shaped by listening to myself—to my heart and soul. Some examples of times that I have *listened* are . . .

Date · Entry

9. Optimal health is a dynamic process, the birthright of *all* beings. My optimal self
    is experienced when I *feel* . . .

Date	Entry

10. Optimal health can be expressed only by a unification of mind, body, and spirit. This is to know the soul within. I experience this state when I am . . .

Date   ·   Entry

No two roads are the same—for our experience is as unique as the footprints we leave behind.

Reflection

We travel so far seeking the secrets of life.

We question and continue to search.

The years pass . . .

Has the mystery revealed itself?

Be still for the universe speaks in silence: listen.

We can now begin to glimpse and know.

*W*hen you take this ultimate journey,
you will rediscover *you* and be astonished
at your ability to touch the core of your being.
With all respect, I invite you to awaken to
the challenge, and transform yourself on
a path of both service and endless joy.

Section D: Actualization of the Ultimate Self

Now, there is a light focused clearly on the road ahead—for some, it may be for the first time. You have obtained true insight into who you really are and where you want to go. This section will help anchor the knowledge of your authentic self as an absolute fact within your being, in case you still have doubts.

The *Appreciative Dialogue* process is again employed. This time you will travel even deeper into your uniqueness to call upon past experiences of elation and celebration. With practice, you will be able to bring peace and harmony to any situation.

Your physicians will probably have all the tables and graphs they need to assess whether your laboratory and therapeutic studies are "normal." But more important to your goal is immediate access to your most intimate aspirations and dreams. This availability is the foremost assurance of the quality of life you seek.

Along the journey many people experience what appears to be a setback. Yet all roads have bends, curves, hills, and an occasional mountain to climb. Remember, any temporary setback is an opportunity to learn. Meanwhile, reconsider the modalities you have chosen, the practitioners involved, or even your primary care physician. If you are satisfied, then perhaps take some time for reflection. Listen closely to your soul—it speaks only in silence.

You are at the crossroads of self-discovery. This is a new beginning to investigate and recognize solutions you never knew possible. To illuminate your path, in the pages that follow comment on the resources, abilities, and expectations you have for yourself today.

1. Desired awareness that I now possess, and resources I've always had . . . .

2. Energetic abilities that I can call upon to sustain optimal health . . . .

3. Therapeutic measures that have assisted me in achieving optimal health . . . .

4. I have obtained optimal health. Therapeutic measures I will participate in to maintain optimal health . . . .

5. I can now identify the living force within my soul and know how best to nurture it.

6. *Integrative protocols* that have changed my life.

7. Optimal health is more than just a *state*; it's the way I experience my life, the way I live *every day*.

8. The enjoyment and pleasure of today is lived to a degree that was unknown only yesterday. "Today is the best it's ever been."

9. I also look forward to tomorrow, for I'm continually growing and becoming my optimal self, the soul to whom I was born.

10. I recognize that *today* is an incredible event, for it encompasses the wisdom of yesterday along with all the possibilities of tomorrow. I can now begin to comprehend my potential and ignite all the passion within.

You will master a methodical thought pattern that allows you to access energetic systems within your own physiology and ignite your body's innate healing properties to obtain optimal health.

Suzanne's Story

Suzanne is a 67-year-old widow who lost her husband almost 25 years ago in a tragic boating accident. The couple had taken pride in the many civic and community organizations in which they participated. They were also a fixture at the local country club and always attended the Winter Ball and all its gala activities. They had no children and thought of the community as their extended family.

However, after the sudden death of her husband, Suzanne became progressively less interested in the outside world and increasingly isolated herself—even from her closest friends. By the summer of 1998, it had been almost 10 years since she had been seen in public. She had become her own prisoner, isolated in her turn-of-the-century Victorian house.

Nearly two years ago, I received a call from her gardener. He had feared "the worst"—that Suzanne had passed on in the night without anyone being alerted. I entered the premises early that morning with the local authorities. To our surprise we found an unkempt, disoriented, older-appearing, but very much alive Suzanne.

It was then that I began visiting her on a biweekly basis. Over the next two years, she received medical, psychological, and spiritual support. After almost eighteen months of intensive therapy, she agreed to participate in *Appreciative Dialogue*. Gradually, she began to see her old friends and even host a monthly luncheon for one of her favorite local charities. Suzanne would not participate in journal writing. The memories, no matter how distant, were just too painful. However, she completed all four sections of *Appreciative Dialogue*, recording her answers on audio tape. We listened to them in silence, and occasionally she would reach for a tissue to wipe away the tears.

On a daily basis, you can find Suzanne in her garden—she has rediscovered her passion for roses! She finds that weekly massages and learning yoga through videotapes ease her sorrow. She also looks forward to monthly acupuncture sessions. She now takes pride in her contributions to community organizations. All of this has rekindled her will to live each day as it comes.

Time is but billions of moments— and if I live each moment well, then I have really lived.

Desired awareness that I now possess, and resources I've always had . . .

Date	Entry
	## *Excerpts from Dr. Tel*

9-3-00 *I acknowledge that my inner healing potential is accessible and allows me to experience an optimal state of health every day.*

My mental state can control my emotional balance and provide positive choices in any situation.

My physical body needs nourishment every day—spiritually, physically, and emotionally.

By being still, I can maximize my healing ability and consciously be aware of my needs.

I enjoy life more by just being aware—this gives me clarity and an opportunity to achieve miracles.

Love is a powerful force . . . I will not miss an opportunity to experience it, to share, or feel the emotion. It is an essential element of optimal well-being.

1. Desired awareness that I now possess, and resources I've always had . . .
    (*Please list resources.*)

Date	Entry

There is nothing that can be said or done to me that would alter my perception
of myself, for my internal focus is a reflection of my soul.

111.

2. Energetic abilities that I can call upon to sustain optimal health . . .

Date · Entry

The most profound changes come from within.

3. Therapeutic measures that have assisted me in achieving optimal health . . .

Date   Entry

4. I have obtained optimal health. Therapeutic measures I will participate in to maintain optimal health . . .

Date	Entry

Our path is often the unconscious mundane; the miracle is instead the road traveled with consciousness in thought, purpose, and deed.

5. I can now identify the living force within my soul and know how best to nurture it. (*Please describe.*)

Date · *Entry*

6. *Integrative protocols* that have changed my life.
    (*Please list.*)

Date	Entry

Look to integrative solutions—their power will amaze you.

7. Optimal health is more than just a *state*; it's the way I experience my life, the way I live *every day*. (*Please describe today.*)

Date   Entry

8. The enjoyment and pleasure of today is lived to a degree that was unknown only yesterday. "Today is the best it's ever been." (*Please explain why.*)

Date	Entry

9. I also look forward to tomorrow, for I'm continually growing and becoming my optimal self, the soul to whom I was born. (*Please comment on your expectations for tomorrow.*)

Date   Entry

10. I recognize that *today* is an incredible event for it encompasses the wisdom of yesterday along with all the possibilities of tomorrow. I can now begin to comprehend my potential and ignite all the passion within. (*Please express yourself.*)

Date · *Entry*

Building healing networks can change our entire society.

Reflection

Allow time to be quiet, to sit in stillness,

to ignore the roar of thoughts that flash

through your conscious mind.

This is the moment of realization.

All is possible in the creation of life's dream.

Your goals are well within your grasp.

Awareness of this moment, this now,

will transform you forever.

Optimal Health Plan

*W*e begin to acknowledge the miracle of life every day and then become able to experience it.

OPTIMAL HEALTH PLAN

The time has come to consolidate the work you have done in Sections A through D. You now have a track record, a path along which you have traveled. However, the road still stretches ahead . . .

It is important to conduct a detailed summary of your healing journey over the recent past. This will facilitate an ongoing dialogue with health professionals, especially your primary care physician.

First, name the proposed therapeutic modalities that you are in the process of trying. What comprises your regimen of treatment, therapy, and remedies? Please complete these portions with the assistance of your physician. Use your experiences thus far as a benchmark for what will come next.

Second, indicate what modalities and treatment options you wish to experience in the future. All the reflecting you have done in your journal can be summarized in these sections. I have provided sample excerpts from my own journey, in which *Appreciative Dialogue* helped to clarify my personal goals and state of mind.

Third, list the choices you eventually plan to try. Be creative in proposing treatment options you believe will enhance your desired outcome. This is a time to imagine the world of possibilities.

Fourth, express the personal solutions you have accomplished on a day-to-day basis and want to include in your overall health plan. For example, I enjoy the practice of daily meditation. It imbues me with balance, peace, and inner strength. Please delight in your own options with the passion of your soul.

Fifth, look ahead without limitation. Now you realize that healing is a quest, not a destination. Dream away to your heart's content—and I do mean *content*.

These five steps that make up your Optimal Health Plan are organized in chart form on the pages that follow and are titled:

Step One: Current Professional Treatment

Step Two: Current Remedies and Supplements

Step Three: Proposed Treatment and Remedies

Step Four: Current Personal Solutions

Step Five: Goals for the Road Ahead

STEP ONE: CURRENT PROFESSIONAL TREATMENT

Please summarize current therapeutic modalities in which you are actively participating. Be specific and keep as current as possible. Think of this as the map of your journey.

Excerpts from Dr. Tel:

| 9-2-00 | Acupuncture/ Chiropractic | Alternate treatments every three months to insure the optimal functioning of my immune and nervous systems. |

Date	Modality	Comments

STEP TWO: CURRENT REMEDIES AND SUPPLEMENTS

Please list all pharmaceuticals (prescriptions, or over-the-counter medicines), supplements (vitamins, herbs, or naturopathic remedies), and any other remedies you are presently taking.

Excerpts from Dr. Tel:

9-2-00	Vit. E 400 i.u.	Daily	Protective antioxidants
	Vit. C 500 mg.	Twice Daily	
		(with breakfast & dinner)	

Name	Dosage	Frequency	Duration	Reason for Taking

STEP THREE: PROPOSED TREATMENT AND REMEDIES

Please indicate the therapeutic modalities and remedies that you would like to try in the future. What do you expect to experience?

Excerpts from Dr. Tel:

9-2-00   Feldenkrais   To be as stretched and toned as my body will allow.

Date	Modality / Remedy	Desired Outcome

STEP FOUR: CURRENT PERSONAL SOLUTIONS

You are now on the path to complete wellness. Optimal health is realistically obtainable.
Please list the personal solutions you have recently tried.

> ### Excerpts from Dr. Tel:
>
> | 9-2-00 | Exercise | I now run / walk every day until my mind is clear and I've reconnected with my soul. |

Date	Solution	Experience

STEP FIVE: GOALS FOR THE ROAD AHEAD

You now realize that healing is a journey, not a destination. You can look ahead and visualize your journey forward to a world of possibilities.

Excerpts from Dr. Tel:

| 9-2-00 | One Year | I awaken in the early morning with the vitality and energy of the rising sun. |

Date	Timeline	Goals
	One Year	
	Five Year	
	Ten Year	
	Fifteen Year	
	Twenty Year	

The Journey Goes On

*H*ave I now come to the end . . . have I "completed" *Appreciative Dialogue*? Does life still start tomorrow? This is the *beginning*, the start of a journey to a world that knows no limitations, where today is dreams yet to be realized. Your reality is now one of possibilities. The choices are endless.

Listening to your heart, come to know the soul that is you and you begin to understand the meaning of life. Discover yourself, and the possibilities within. Welcome to the *beginning* and celebrate the journey.

I know how to
create the life
I desire.

THE JOURNEY GOES ON

By now, you have probably realized that this book—your journey—
is about more than health or any particular illness or imbalance you may
face. Regardless of the situation, there can be no separation between you
and what you are feeling. It is through this willingness to *feel* that you
meet your total self. In return, you generate dynamic solutions and
synergistic relationships leading to inner harmony, balance, and optimal
health.

When you sense beyond the physical body, you merge with your
multi-dimensional self: a soul, a spirit, and a creative instinct at the seat of
energetic systems. This inner place of truth knows nothing of doubt or
fear. Anchored at the center, you are set firmly on the path of self-
discovery, destined for better, more conscious choices. The world
becomes a huge menu of opportunity and your mind explodes with
unlimited genius.

Also of importance is your relationship with each of the partners who
will guide you along the way. Perhaps by now you have completed your
journal and shared it with your physician. This is your primary health care
partner, whose help is key to creating an effective overall plan for your
specific needs. In addition, I urge you to seek out complementary
professionals who are willing to dialogue: doctors, chiropractors, holistic
health care professionals, and so on.

Finding your partners may prove challenging at first because many
physicians are not yet familiar with *Appreciative Dialogue*. To help them
become acquainted with this method, I suggest an approach using
openness, clarity, and patience. Soon, your health care guides will be
amazed at your progress from this program.

The dialogue will ignite your imagination and access vital energy forces—there will be no limit. And, by evaluating your responses to the questions, you reinforce a newfound perspective. This is a lifelong creative process of eliciting what has been heretofore unfelt or unknown, then using it to manifest something wonderful.

Learning any new skill takes time and commitment, whether it is flying a plane or training for a marathon. Moreover, it requires courage to follow the unfamiliar while being totally comfortable with who you are becoming—the essence of your self, the unique person you already are! For these tasks, you will need an unconditional support team—family, friends, and caring groups. Of course, some people are more able to help than others. But everyone contributes something to putting together your life "puzzle." Thus, sharing experiences with others is an essential part of the journey.

What is beautiful about *Appreciative Dialogue* is that it serves EVERYONE—patients, health care providers, and supporters alike. Once people agree to interact with you, they will experience a similar evolution and fulfillment in their own lives. Eventually, such support systems will connect on larger levels to form integrative healing networks across the nation. It is my vision that by the *Autumn of 2002,* we will have the first of these networks in place. They will foster a broad spectrum of treatment options, unified in all aspects of health care, to insure the experience of optimal healing and well-being.

Appreciative Dialogue is about the opportunity for conscious decision making without limitations. There is no "right" path. But by seeking solutions we are guided on our own unique journey. I sincerely hope your journey brings the ultimate that life has to offer and the peace your soul desires. Together we can dramatically change ours to a world where dreams indeed come true. I welcome comments about the adventures you have encountered in the realization of your own miracles.

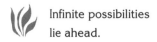 Infinite possibilities lie ahead.

Reflection

Expect a Miracle will enrich every aspect
of your life as it nourishes your soul.
All who are touched will be forever changed.
Listen to your heart, come to know the soul that is you.
Discover the truth that lies within and celebrate your life!

Addenda & Suggested Reading

In the following pages I have included Addenda A and B as referred to in the text.

The Physician Letter is a generic format that may be useful in the initial phase of finding your primary care physician.

The Treatment Summary is a helpful summary to share with your health care providers and to recap your optimal health plan.

A list of books for suggested reading follows, to assist in your own understanding about treatment options and approaches.

Addendum A
Introductory Letter to Physician

Date: _____

Dear Dr. _____,

I have just completed *Expect a Miracle . . . You Won't Be Disappointed!* by Tel Franklin, M.D.

I'm planning to begin *Appreciative Dialogue* on _____ [date]. This is a four-part journal in which I participate in exploring both conventional and alternative medical modalities.

The reason I have chosen this program is:

I would like to schedule an introductory visit and assessment to share the journal questions and format. I hope that you will consider partnering with me on this journey.

Thank you for your time and consideration.

Sincerely,

Addendum B
Treatment Summary

    Before beginning each treatment modality, comment on your perceived expectations. After each experience, comment on the effects: physical, psychological, and spiritual. Be specific about how you see the treatment fitting into your overall healing journey.

Modality / Provider	Met Expectations	Exceeded Expectations	Comments

[continued]

Addendum B
Treatment Summary

[continued]

Modality / Provider	Met Expectations	Exceeded Expectations	Comments

Suggested Reading

Anselmo, Peter with James S. Brooks, M.D. 1996. Ayurvedic secrets to longevity and total health. Paramus, NJ: Prentice Hall.

Beinfield, Harriet, L.Ac. and Efrem Korngold, L.Ac., O.M.D. 1991. Between heaven and earth: A guide to Chinese medicine. New York: Ballantine.

Bloomfield, Harold, M.D. 1998. Healing anxiety with herbs. New York: Harper Collins.

Brennan, Richard. 1991. Alexander technique: Natural poise for health. Rockport, MA: Element.

Castleman, Michael. 2000. Blended medicine: The best choices in healing. Emmaus, PA: Rodale.

Carnie, L.V. 1998. Chi gung. St. Paul, MN: Llewellyn.

Chodron, Pema. 1991. The wisdom of no escape. Boston: Shambhala

Chopra, Deepak, M.D. 1994. The seven spiritual laws of success: A practical guide to the fulfillment of your dreams. Novato and San Rafael, CA: New World Library/ Amber-Allen.

Cohen, Kenneth. 1997. The way of qi gong: The art and science of Chinese energy healing. New York: Ballantine.

Dalai Lama, His Holiness the. 1999. Ethics for the new millennium. New York: Riverhead Books.

Dossey, Larry, M.D. 1997. Prayer is good medicine: How to reap the healing benefits of prayer. New York: Harper Collins.

Dossey, Larry, M.D. 1999. Reinventing medicine: Beyond mind-body to a new era of healing. New York: Harper Collins.

Gerber, Richard, M.D. 2000. Vibrational medicine for the 21st century: The complete guide to energy healing and spiritual transformation. New York: Eagle Brook/ Harper Collins.

Goldberg, Burton et al., compilers. 1993. Alternative Medicine: The definitive guide. Puyallup, WA: Future Medicine.

Gordon, Richard. 1999. Quantum touch: The power to heal. Berkeley, CA: North Atlantic Books.

Kaptchuk, Ted, O.M.D. 1983. The web that has no weaver: Understanding Chinese medicine. Chicago: Congdon & Weed.

Lambert, Mary with Chris Parks, usui master. 2000. An introduction to Reiki. London: Collins & Brown.

Morton, Mary and Michael Morton. 2000. Five steps to selecting the best alternative medicine: A guide to complementary and integrated health care. Novato, CA: New World Library.

Myss, Caroline, Ph.D. and C. Norman Shealy, M.D. 1993. The creation of health: The emotional, psychological, and spiritual responses that promote health and healing. New York: Three Rivers Press.

Murray, Michael. 1995. The healing power of herbs. Rocklin, CA: Prima.

Murray, Michael and Joseph Pizzorno. 1998. Encyclopedia of natural medicine. Rocklin, CA: Prima.

Rami, Swami, Rudolph Ballentine, M.D., and Alan Hymes, M.D. 1979, 1998. Science of breath. Honesdale, PA: Himalayan Institute Press.

Reid, Daniel. 1998. A complete guide to chi-gung. Boston: Shambhala.

Ruiz, Don Miguel. 1997. The four agreements: A practical guide to personal freedom. San Rafael, CA: Amber-Allen.

Santorelli, Saki. 1999. Heal thyself: Lessons on mindfulness in medicine. New York: Bell Tower.

Schiller, David and Carol Schiller. 1996. Aromatherapy for mind and body. New York: Sterling.

Serizawa, Katsusuke i Tsubo. 1976. Vital points for oriental therapy. Tokyo: Japan Publications.

Shealy, C. Norman, M.D. 1999. The complete illustrated encyclopedia of alternative healing therapies. Boston: Element.

Siegel, Bernie, M.D. 1990. Love, medicine & miracles: Lessons learned about self-healing from a surgeon's experience with exceptional patients. New York: Harper Collins.

Smith, Randy. 1997. Diagnosis unknown: Our journey to an unconventional cure. Charlottesville, VA: Hampton Roads.

Tiwari, Maya. 1995. Ayurveda: Secrets of healing. Twin Lakes, WI: Lotus Press.

Tolle, Eckhart. 1999. The power of now: A guide to spiritual enlightenment. Novato, CA: New World Library.

Weil, Andrew, M.D. 1995. Spontaneous healing. New York: Ballantine.

Zi, Nancy. 1997. The art of breathing. Six simple lessons to improve performance, health, and well-being. Glendale, CA: Vivi Company.

Zukav, Gary. 2000. Soul stories. New York: Simon & Schuster.

A note from Tel Franklin

I encourage you to share your experiences of *Appreciative Dialogue* with all those around you—and with us.

We are presently building an organization to construct multi-specialty groups for the purpose of creating optimal change for all those seeking the ultimate journey: to fulfill all the hopes and dreams of healthy and creative living every day.

Please contact us:

CENTER FOR APPRECIATIVE DIALOGUE

335 El Dorado Street, Suite 6
Monterey, California 93940
www.AppreciativeDialogue.org

About The Author

Tel Franklin, M.D., is a Board-certified physician and a Fellow of the American Academy of Family Physicians. Dr. Franklin also holds advanced degrees in chemistry and medicine. He completed graduate medical studies at East Carolina University and trained at The London Hospital Medical College, University of London. He is credentialed in Medical Acupuncture through the University of California at Los Angeles, School of Medicine, and has completed advanced study in Traditional Chinese Medicine.

At the University Health Systems of Eastern Carolina, Dr. Franklin authored and was the primary investigator for studies on treating coronary heart disease through lifestyle modifications. As an experienced educator, he has presented seminars and workshops and has been a guest speaker at major medical conventions. He has been awarded many honors for academic, scholastic, and research achievements.

Dr. Franklin integrates Eastern and Western philosophy. He has created an individualized approach to patient care that is solution-driven. When patients and practitioners enter a partnership in healing, they generate positive, creative solutions. He is in private practice and lives on the Monterey Peninsula in California.

ACKNOWLEDGEMENT

I wish to thank Kedron Bryson whose organizational skills allow function and structure to merge. I am grateful for her intellect and passion, and most of all her gift of creative instinct.

Thanks to Ann West for her editorial expertise. It is guided by her wisdom and truly gifted spirit.

Michaelia Morgan and Becky Schilling bring clarity to this project, a vision of a world and the realization of the ultimate journey.

Dr. Tel Franklin offers a vision of health care that empowers the patient and redefines the patient-physician relationship as a *partnership*. It is contemporary health care in its purest form. This solution-driven approach creates integrative protocols and will spur the creation of healing networks across the country.

Dr. Franklin is available for seminars, workshops, or as a keynote speaker.